FitLiber

Fitness & Workout Log/Diary

2014

FitLiber, Fitness & Workout Log/Diary

ISBN-13: 978-1502463579
ISBN-10: 1502463571

Illustrations credit: www.freepik.com

Contents

Info

Name ....

Surname ....

Phone ....

E-mail ....

Height ....   Body fat % (BF).............................

Weight.......................................   Body mass index (BMI) ....

Size (radius)

Neck ....

Chest...

Arms

Waist..

Wrist ....

Hips..

Forearm ....

Thighs ....

Upper arm ....

Calf..

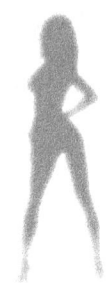

Maximum

	Pull-up	Squat	Deadlift
max.			

	Bench Press		
max.			

max.			

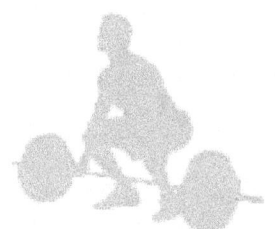

Goals

3 months

....

....

....

....

....

....

....

....

....

....

....

....

....

....

....

....

....

6 months

....
....
....
....
....
....
....
....
....
....
....
....
....
....
....
....
....
....
....

9 months

....
....
....
....
....
....
....
....
....
....
....
....
....
....
....
....
....

12 months

....
....
....
....
....
....
....
....
....
....
....
....
....
....
....
....
....
....

Monthly Progress

Size (radius)

	Weight	Neck	Wrist	Forearm	Upper arm	Chest	Waist	Hips	Thighs	Calf	BF(%)	BMI
January												
February												
March												
April												
May												
June												
July												
August												
September												
October												
November												
December												

Maximum

	Pull-up	Squat	Deadlift	Bench press					
January									
February									
March									
April									
May									
June									
July									
August									
September									
October									
November									
December									

Miscellaneous

January							
February							
March							
April							
May							
June							
July							
August							
September							
October							
November							
December							

Comments

....
....
....
....
....
....
....
....
....
....
....
....
....
....
....

WORKOUTS

WORKOUT ....   Date............................

Exercise	Sets	Reps	Weight	PR

Cardio	Time	Distance	Intensity	PR

Supplements...
....

Comments ....
....
....

things to improve .... things to try out.................................
....

WORKOUT ....   Date..............................

Exercise	Sets	Reps	Weight	PR

Cardio	Time	Distance	Intensity	PR

Supplements..
....

Comments ....
....
....

things to improve ....   things to try out..
....

WORKOUT .... Date...

Exercise	Sets	Reps	Weight	PR

Cardio	Time	Distance	Intensity	PR

Supplements...
....

Comments ....
....
....

things to improve .... things to try out...
....

WORKOUT ....   Date.................................

Exercise	Sets	Reps	Weight	PR

Cardio	Time	Distance	Intensity	PR

Supplements...
....

Comments ....
....
....

things to improve ....   things to try out...
....

WORKOUT ....   Date................................

Exercise	Sets	Reps	Weight	PR

Cardio	Time	Distance	Intensity	PR

Supplements..
....

Comments ....
....
....

things to improve ....   things to try out.............................
....

WORKOUT .... Date...

Exercise	Sets	Reps	Weight	PR

Cardio	Time	Distance	Intensity	PR

Supplements...
....

Comments ....
....
....

things to improve .... things to try out...
....

WORKOUT .... Date.................................

Exercise	Sets	Reps	Weight	PR

Cardio	Time	Distance	Intensity	PR

Supplements..
....

Comments ....
....
....

things to improve ....   things to try out..
....

WORKOUT ....   Date...................................

Exercise	Sets	Reps	Weight	PR

Cardio	Time	Distance	Intensity	PR

Supplements...
....

Comments ....
....
....

things to improve ....   things to try out...
....

WORKOUT .... Date..................................

Exercise	Sets	Reps	Weight	PR

Cardio	Time	Distance	Intensity	PR

Supplements..
....

Comments ....
....
....

things to improve .... things to try out.............................
....

WORKOUT ....   Date...

Exercise	Sets	Reps	Weight	PR

Cardio	Time	Distance	Intensity	PR

Supplements...
....

Comments ....
....
....

things to improve ....   things to try out...
....

WORKOUT .... Date...

Exercise	Sets	Reps	Weight	PR

Cardio	Time	Distance	Intensity	PR

Supplements..

....

Comments ....

....

....

things to improve .... things to try out..

....

WORKOUT ....   Date................................

Exercise	Sets	Reps	Weight	PR

Cardio	Time	Distance	Intensity	PR

Supplements...
....

Comments ....
....
....

things to improve ....   things to try out...
....

WORKOUT .... Date..................................

Exercise	Sets	Reps	Weight	PR

Cardio	Time	Distance	Intensity	PR

Supplements...

....

Comments ....

....

....

things to improve .... things to try out...

....

WORKOUT .... Date ....

Exercise	Sets	Reps	Weight	PR

Cardio	Time	Distance	Intensity	PR

Supplements ....
....

Comments ....
....
....

things to improve .... things to try out ....
....

WORKOUT .... Date..

Exercise	Sets	Reps	Weight	PR

Cardio	Time	Distance	Intensity	PR

Supplements...
....

Comments ....
....
....

things to improve .... things to try out..
....

WORKOUT ....   Date...................................

Exercise	Sets	Reps	Weight	PR

Cardio	Time	Distance	Intensity	PR

Supplements..
....

Comments ....
....
....

things to improve ....   things to try out...
....

WORKOUT .... Date..................................

Exercise	Sets	Reps	Weight	PR

Cardio	Time	Distance	Intensity	PR

Supplements...

....

Comments ....

....

....

things to improve .... things to try out...

....

WORKOUT ....   Date.................................

Exercise	Sets	Reps	Weight	PR

Cardio	Time	Distance	Intensity	PR

Supplements...
....

Comments ....
....
....

things to improve ....   things to try out...................................
....

WORKOUT .... Date ....

Exercise	Sets	Reps	Weight	PR

Cardio	Time	Distance	Intensity	PR

Supplements ....

....

Comments ....

....

....

things to improve .... things to try out ....

....

WORKOUT ....   Date...................................

Exercise	Sets	Reps	Weight	PR

Cardio	Time	Distance	Intensity	PR

Supplements...
....

Comments ....
....
....

things to improve ....   things to try out.................................
....

WORKOUT .... Date...

Exercise	Sets	Reps	Weight	PR

Cardio	Time	Distance	Intensity	PR

Supplements...
....

Comments ....
....
....

things to improve ....   things to try out..
....

WORKOUT ....   Date...................................

Exercise	Sets	Reps	Weight	PR

Cardio	Time	Distance	Intensity	PR

Supplements..
....

Comments ....
....
....

things to improve ....   things to try out..
....

WORKOUT .... Date..

Exercise	Sets	Reps	Weight	PR

Cardio	Time	Distance	Intensity	PR

Supplements...
....

Comments ....
....
....

things to improve .... things to try out...
....

WORKOUT ....   Date.................................

Exercise	Sets	Reps	Weight	PR

Cardio	Time	Distance	Intensity	PR

Supplements...
....

Comments ....
....
....

things to improve ....   things to try out...................................
....

WORKOUT ....   Date...

Exercise	Sets	Reps	Weight	PR

Cardio	Time	Distance	Intensity	PR

Supplements...
....

Comments ....
....
....

things to improve ....   things to try out ....
....

WORKOUT ....   Date......................................

Exercise	Sets	Reps	Weight	PR

Cardio	Time	Distance	Intensity	PR

Supplements...

....

Comments ....

....

....

things to improve ....   things to try out...

....

WORKOUT .... Date ....

Exercise	Sets	Reps	Weight	PR

Cardio	Time	Distance	Intensity	PR

Supplements ....
....

Comments ....
....
....

things to improve .... things to try out ....
....

WORKOUT .... Date..................................

Exercise	Sets	Reps	Weight	PR

Cardio	Time	Distance	Intensity	PR

Supplements...
....

Comments ....
....
....

things to improve .... things to try out...................................
....

WORKOUT .... Date...................................

Exercise	Sets	Reps	Weight	PR

Cardio	Time	Distance	Intensity	PR

Supplements...
....

Comments ....
....
....

things to improve ....   things to try out...........................
....

WORKOUT .... Date................................

Exercise	Sets	Reps	Weight	PR

Cardio	Time	Distance	Intensity	PR

Supplements..
....

Comments ....
....
....

things to improve .... things to try out...
....

WORKOUT .... Date...

Exercise	Sets	Reps	Weight	PR

Cardio	Time	Distance	Intensity	PR

Supplements...
....

Comments ....
....
....

things to improve .... things to try out..
....

WORKOUT ....   Date..

Exercise	Sets	Reps	Weight	PR

Cardio	Time	Distance	Intensity	PR

Supplements..
....

Comments ....
....
....

things to improve ....   things to try out...
....

WORKOUT .... Date................................

Exercise	Sets	Reps	Weight	PR

Cardio	Time	Distance	Intensity	PR

Supplements...
....

Comments ....
....
....

things to improve .... things to try out................................
....

WORKOut ....   Date...

Exercise	Sets	Reps	Weight	PR

Cardio	Time	Distance	Intensity	PR

Supplements...
....

Comments ....
....
....

things to improve ....   things to try out...
....

WORKOUT ....   Date..

Exercise	Sets	Reps	Weight	PR

Cardio	Time	Distance	Intensity	PR

Supplements..
....

Comments ....
....
....

things to improve ....   things to try out..
....

WORKOUT ....   Date..

Exercise	Sets	Reps	Weight	PR

Cardio	Time	Distance	Intensity	PR

Supplements...
....

Comments ....
....
....

things to improve ....   things to try out...
....

WORKOUT .... Date...................................

Exercise	Sets	Reps	Weight	PR

Cardio	Time	Distance	Intensity	PR

Supplements...
....

Comments ....
....
....

things to improve .... things to try out...
....

WorKout ....   Date.................................

Exercise	Sets	Reps	Weight	PR

Cardio	Time	Distance	Intensity	PR

Supplements...
....

Comments ....
....
....

things to improve ....   things to try out.................................
....

WORKOUT .... Date...

Exercise	Sets	Reps	Weight	PR

Cardio	Time	Distance	Intensity	PR

Supplements..
....

Comments ....
....
....

things to improve .... things to try out...
....

WORKOUT ....   Date.................................

Exercise	Sets	Reps	Weight	PR

Cardio	Time	Distance	Intensity	PR

Supplements...
....

Comments ....
....
....

things to improve ....   things to try out..
....

WORKOUT .... Date...

Exercise	Sets	Reps	Weight	PR

Cardio	Time	Distance	Intensity	PR

Supplements...
....

Comments ....
....
....

things to improve .... things to try out...
....

WORKOUT ....   Date.......................................

Exercise	Sets	Reps	Weight	PR

Cardio	Time	Distance	Intensity	PR

Supplements...
....

Comments ....
....
....

things to improve ....   things to try out...............................
....

WORKOUT ....   Date...

Exercise	Sets	Reps	Weight	PR

Cardio	Time	Distance	Intensity	PR

Supplements..

....

Comments ....

....

....

things to improve .... things to try out...

....

WORKOUT .... Date ....

Exercise	Sets	Reps	Weight	PR

Cardio	Time	Distance	Intensity	PR

Supplements ....
....

Comments ....
....
....

things to improve .... things to try out ....
....

WORKOUT .... Date....................................

Exercise	Sets	Reps	Weight	PR

Cardio	Time	Distance	Intensity	PR

Supplements...

....

Comments ....

....

....

things to improve .... things to try out...

....

WORKOUT .... Date...............................

Exercise	Sets	Reps	Weight	PR

Cardio	Time	Distance	Intensity	PR

Supplements..
....

Comments ....
....
....

things to improve ....   things to try out.....................................
....

WORKOUT .... Date..................................

Exercise	Sets	Reps	Weight	PR

Cardio	Time	Distance	Intensity	PR

Supplements...
....

Comments ....
....
....

things to improve .... things to try out...
....

WORKOUT .... Date...............................

Exercise	Sets	Reps	Weight	PR

Cardio	Time	Distance	Intensity	PR

Supplements...
....

Comments ....
....
....

things to improve ....   things to try out...
....

WORKOUT .... Date...

Exercise	Sets	Reps	Weight	PR

Cardio	Time	Distance	Intensity	PR

Supplements..
....

Comments ....
....
....

things to improve .... things to try out......................................
....

WORKOUT ....   Date................................

Exercise	Sets	Reps	Weight	PR

Cardio	Time	Distance	Intensity	PR

Supplements...
....

Comments ....
....
....

things to improve ....   things to try out...
....

WORKOUT .... Date ....

Exercise	Sets	Reps	Weight	PR

Cardio	Time	Distance	Intensity	PR

Supplements ....
....

Comments ....
....
....

things to improve .... things to try out ....
....

WORKOUT .... Date....................................

Exercise	Sets	Reps	Weight	PR

Cardio	Time	Distance	Intensity	PR

Supplements..
....

Comments ....
....
....

things to improve .... things to try out...................................
....

WORKOUT .... Date...

Exercise	Sets	Reps	Weight	PR

Cardio	Time	Distance	Intensity	PR

Supplements..

....

Comments ....

....

....

things to improve .... things to try out...

....

WORKOUT .... Date....................................

Exercise	Sets	Reps	Weight	PR

Cardio	Time	Distance	Intensity	PR

Supplements...
....

Comments ....
....
....

things to improve ....   things to try out.......................................
....

WORKOUT .... Date...

Exercise	Sets	Reps	Weight	PR

Cardio	Time	Distance	Intensity	PR

Supplements...
....

Comments ....
....
....

things to improve .... things to try out...
....

WORKOUT .... Date..

Exercise	Sets	Reps	Weight	PR

Cardio	Time	Distance	Intensity	PR

Supplements...
....

Comments ....
....
....

things to improve .... things to try out ....
....

WORKOUT .... Date...

Exercise	Sets	Reps	Weight	PR

Cardio	Time	Distance	Intensity	PR

Supplements..
....

Comments ....
....
....

things to improve .... things to try out...
....

WORKOUT ....   Date.......................................

Exercise	Sets	Reps	Weight	PR

Cardio	Time	Distance	Intensity	PR

Supplements...
....

Comments ....
....
....

things to improve ....   things to try out...
....

WORKOUT .... Date...

Exercise	Sets	Reps	Weight	PR

Cardio	Time	Distance	Intensity	PR

Supplements...
....

Comments ....
....
....

things to improve .... things to try out...
....

WORKOUT ....   Date.................................

Exercise	Sets	Reps	Weight	PR

Cardio	Time	Distance	Intensity	PR

Supplements...
....

Comments ....
....
....

things to improve ....   things to try out...
....

WORKOUT .... Date.......................................

Exercise	Sets	Reps	Weight	PR

Cardio	Time	Distance	Intensity	PR

Supplements...

....

Comments ....

....

....

things to improve .... things to try out..

....

WORKOUT .... Date..................................

Exercise	Sets	Reps	Weight	PR

Cardio	Time	Distance	Intensity	PR

Supplements...
....

Comments ....
....
....

things to improve .... things to try out...
....

WORKOUT .... Date..................................

Exercise	Sets	Reps	Weight	PR

Cardio	Time	Distance	Intensity	PR

Supplements...

....

Comments ....

....

....

things to improve .... things to try out................................

....

WORKOUT ....   Date....................................

Exercise	Sets	Reps	Weight	PR

Cardio	Time	Distance	Intensity	PR

Supplements..
....

Comments ....
....
....

things to improve ....   things to try out..............................
....

WORKOUT .... Date..................................

Exercise	Sets	Reps	Weight	PR

Cardio	Time	Distance	Intensity	PR

Supplements..
....

Comments ....
....
....

things to improve .... things to try out...................................
....

Workout .... Date...................................

Exercise	Sets	Reps	Weight	PR

Cardio	Time	Distance	Intensity	PR

Supplements..
....

Comments ....
....
....

things to improve .... things to try out...................................
....

WORKOUT ....   Date...

Exercise	Sets	Reps	Weight	PR

Cardio	Time	Distance	Intensity	PR

supplements...
....

Comments ....
....
....

things to improve ....   things to try out...
....

WORKOUT ....   Date..

Exercise	Sets	Reps	Weight	PR

Cardio	Time	Distance	Intensity	PR

Supplements...
....

Comments ....
....
....

things to improve ....   things to try out.......................................
....

WORKOUT ....   Date....................................

Exercise	Sets	Reps	Weight	PR

Cardio	Time	Distance	Intensity	PR

Supplements...
....

Comments ....
....
....

things to improve ....   things to try out...
....

WORKOUT .... Date...............................

Exercise	Sets	Reps	Weight	PR

Cardio	Time	Distance	Intensity	PR

Supplements...
....

Comments ....
....
....

things to improve .... things to try out...........................
....

WORKOUT .... Date....................................

Exercise	Sets	Reps	Weight	PR

Cardio	Time	Distance	Intensity	PR

Supplements..
....

Comments ....
....
....

things to improve .... things to try out.................................
....

WORKOUT ....   Date.................................

Exercise	Sets	Reps	Weight	PR

Cardio	Time	Distance	Intensity	PR

Supplements...
....

Comments ....
....
....

things to improve ....   things to try out.................................
....

WORKOUT .... Date..................................

Exercise	Sets	Reps	Weight	PR

Cardio	Time	Distance	Intensity	PR

Supplements...

....

Comments ....

....

....

things to improve .... things to try out...

....

WORKOUT .... Date................................

Exercise	Sets	Reps	Weight	PR

Cardio	Time	Distance	Intensity	PR

Supplements...
....

Comments ....
....
....

things to improve ....   things to try out..................................
....

WORKOUT .... Date ....

Exercise	Sets	Reps	Weight	PR

Cardio	Time	Distance	Intensity	PR

Supplements ....
....

Comments ....
....
....

things to improve .... things to try out ....
....

Workout ....   Date ....

Exercise	Sets	Reps	Weight	PR

Cardio	Time	Distance	Intensity	PR

Supplements ....
....

Comments ....
....
....

things to improve ....   things to try out ....
....

WORKOUT ....   Date...

Exercise	Sets	Reps	Weight	PR

Cardio	Time	Distance	Intensity	PR

Supplements...
....

Comments ....
....
....

things to improve .... things to try out...
....

WORKOUT ....   Date...............................

Exercise	Sets	Reps	Weight	PR

Cardio	Time	Distance	Intensity	PR

Supplements...
....

Comments ....
....
....

things to improve ....   things to try out.................................
....

WORKOUT .... Date ....

Exercise	Sets	Reps	Weight	PR

Cardio	Time	Distance	Intensity	PR

Supplements ....
....

Comments ....
....
....

things to improve .... things to try out ....
....

WORKOUT ....   Date..

Exercise	Sets	Reps	Weight	PR

Cardio	Time	Distance	Intensity	PR

Supplements...
....

Comments ....
....
....

things to improve ....   things to try out...
....

WORKOUT ....   Date.................................

Exercise	Sets	Reps	Weight	PR

Cardio	Time	Distance	Intensity	PR

Supplements..
....

Comments ....
....
....

things to improve ....   things to try out...
....

WORKOUT ....   Date.......................................

Exercise	Sets	Reps	Weight	PR

Cardio	Time	Distance	Intensity	PR

Supplements...
....

Comments ....
....
....

things to improve ....   things to try out...
....

WORKOUT ....   Date.................................

Exercise	Sets	Reps	Weight	PR

Cardio	Time	Distance	Intensity	PR

Supplements...
....

Comments ....
....
....

things to improve ....   things to try out.................................
....

WORKOUT ....   Date.....................................

Exercise	Sets	Reps	Weight	PR

Cardio	Time	Distance	Intensity	PR

Supplements...
....

Comments ....
....
....

things to improve ....   things to try out...
....

WORKOUT .... Date............................

Exercise	Sets	Reps	Weight	PR

Cardio	Time	Distance	Intensity	PR

Supplements..
....

Comments ....
....
....

things to improve .... things to try out..
....

WORKOUT .... Date...............................

Exercise	Sets	Reps	Weight	PR

Cardio	Time	Distance	Intensity	PR

Supplements..
....

Comments ....
....
....

things to improve ....   things to try out..
....

WORKOUT .... Date.................................

Exercise	Sets	Reps	Weight	PR

Cardio	Time	Distance	Intensity	PR

Supplements...
....

Comments ....
....
....

things to improve ....   things to try out.............................
....

WORKOUT ....   Date...........................

Exercise	Sets	Reps	Weight	PR

Cardio	Time	Distance	Intensity	PR

Supplements..
....

Comments ....
....
....

things to improve ....   things to try out...
....

WORKOUT ....   Date..................................

Exercise	Sets	Reps	Weight	PR

Cardio	Time	Distance	Intensity	PR

Supplements...
....

Comments ....
....
....

things to improve ....   things to try out...
....

WORKOUT ....   Date..

Exercise	Sets	Reps	Weight	PR

Cardio	Time	Distance	Intensity	PR

Supplements...
....

Comments ....
....
....

things to improve ....   things to try out...
....

WORKOUT ....   Date..

Exercise	Sets	Reps	Weight	PR

Cardio	Time	Distance	Intensity	PR

Supplements...
....

Comments ....
....
....

things to improve ....   things to try out..
....

Workout ....   Date.......................................

Exercise	Sets	Reps	Weight	PR

Cardio	Time	Distance	Intensity	PR

Supplements..
....

Comments ....
....
....

things to improve ....   things to try out.......................................
....

WORKOUT .... Date..

Exercise	Sets	Reps	Weight	PR

Cardio	Time	Distance	Intensity	PR

Supplements..
....

Comments ....
....
....

things to improve .... things to try out...
....

WORKOUT ....   Date.....................................

Exercise	Sets	Reps	Weight	PR

Cardio	Time	Distance	Intensity	PR

Supplements...
....

Comments ....
....
....

things to improve ....   things to try out...
....

WORKOUT .... Date.....................................

Exercise	Sets	Reps	Weight	PR

Cardio	Time	Distance	Intensity	PR

Supplements...
....

Comments ....
....
....

things to improve .... things to try out...
....

WORKOUT ....   Date..............................

Exercise	Sets	Reps	Weight	PR

Cardio	Time	Distance	Intensity	PR

Supplements..
....

Comments ....
....
....

things to improve ....   things to try out...
....

WORKOUT .... Date ....

Exercise	Sets	Reps	Weight	PR

Cardio	Time	Distance	Intensity	PR

Supplements ....
....

Comments ....
....
....

things to improve ....   things to try out ....
....

WORKOUT .... Date................................

Exercise	Sets	Reps	Weight	PR

Cardio	Time	Distance	Intensity	PR

Supplements...
....

Comments ....
....
....

things to improve .... things to try out..
....

WORKOUT .... Date..

Exercise	Sets	Reps	Weight	PR

Cardio	Time	Distance	Intensity	PR

Supplements...
....

Comments ....
....
....

things to improve .... things to try out.......................................
....

WORKOUT ....   Date.................................

Exercise	Sets	Reps	Weight	PR

Cardio	Time	Distance	Intensity	PR

Supplements...
....

Comments ....
....
....

things to improve ....   things to try out.....................................
....

WORKOUT .... Date...

Exercise	Sets	Reps	Weight	PR

Cardio	Time	Distance	Intensity	PR

Supplements...
....

Comments ....
....
....

things to improve .... things to try out...
....

WORKOUT ....   Date.......................................

Exercise	Sets	Reps	Weight	PR

Cardio	Time	Distance	Intensity	PR

Supplements...
....

Comments ....
....
....

things to improve ....   things to try out...................................
....

WORKOUT .... Date................................

Exercise	Sets	Reps	Weight	PR

Cardio	Time	Distance	Intensity	PR

Supplements..
....

Comments ....
....
....

things to improve .... things to try out..................................
....

WORKOUT ....   Date..................................

Exercise	Sets	Reps	Weight	PR

Cardio	Time	Distance	Intensity	PR

Supplements..
....

Comments ....
....
....

things to improve ....   things to try out...................................
....

WORKOUT ....   Date........................

Exercise	Sets	Reps	Weight	PR

Cardio	Time	Distance	Intensity	PR

Supplements..
....

Comments ....
....
....

things to improve ....   things to try out..............................
....

WORKOUT .... Date...................................

Exercise	Sets	Reps	Weight	PR

Cardio	Time	Distance	Intensity	PR

Supplements...
....

Comments ....
....
....

things to improve ....   things to try out...
....

WORKOUT .... Date...

Exercise	Sets	Reps	Weight	PR

Cardio	Time	Distance	Intensity	PR

Supplements...
....

Comments ....
....
....

things to improve .... things to try out...
....

WORKOUT ....   Date.................................

Exercise	Sets	Reps	Weight	PR

Cardio	Time	Distance	Intensity	PR

Supplements..
....

Comments ....
....
....

things to improve ....   things to try out.................................
....

Workout ....   Date................................

Exercise	Sets	Reps	Weight	PR

Cardio	Time	Distance	Intensity	PR

Supplements..
....

Comments ....
....
....

things to improve ....   things to try out...................................
....

WORKOUT ....   Date...................................

Exercise	Sets	Reps	Weight	PR

Cardio	Time	Distance	Intensity	PR

Supplements...
....

Comments ....
....
....

things to improve ....   things to try out.................................
....

WORKOUT .... Date..

Exercise	Sets	Reps	Weight	PR

Cardio	Time	Distance	Intensity	PR

Supplements...
....

Comments ....
....
....

things to improve .... things to try out...
....

WORKOUT ....   Date..................................

Exercise	Sets	Reps	Weight	PR

Cardio	Time	Distance	Intensity	PR

Supplements...
....

Comments ....
....
....

things to improve ....   things to try out....................................
....

WORKOUT ....   Date..................................

Exercise	Sets	Reps	Weight	PR

Cardio	Time	Distance	Intensity	PR

Supplements...

....

Comments ....

....

....

things to improve ....   things to try out....................................

....

Workout .... Date.......................................

Exercise	Sets	Reps	Weight	PR

Cardio	Time	Distance	Intensity	PR

Supplements..
....

Comments ....
....
....

things to improve .... things to try out..................................
....

WORKOUT .... Date...

Exercise	Sets	Reps	Weight	PR

Cardio	Time	Distance	Intensity	PR

Supplements..
....

Comments ....
....
....

things to improve .... things to try out.......................................
....

WORKOUT

Workout .... Date ....

Exercise	Sets	Reps	Weight	PR

Cardio	Time	Distance	Intensity	PR

Supplements ....
....

Comments ....
....
....

things to improve .... things to try out ....
....

WORKOUT .... Date...

Exercise	Sets	Reps	Weight	PR

Cardio	Time	Distance	Intensity	PR

Supplements...
....

Comments ....
....
....

things to improve .... things to try out...
....

WORKOUT .... Date..................................

Exercise	Sets	Reps	Weight	PR

Cardio	Time	Distance	Intensity	PR

Supplements..
....

Comments ....
....
....

things to improve .... things to try out................................
....

WORKOUT .... Date..

Exercise	Sets	Reps	Weight	PR

Cardio	Time	Distance	Intensity	PR

Supplements...
....

Comments ....
....
....

things to improve .... things to try out..
....

WORKOUT ....   Date.................................

Exercise	Sets	Reps	Weight	PR

Cardio	Time	Distance	Intensity	PR

Supplements..
....

Comments ....
....
....

things to improve ....   things to try out...................................
....

WORKOUT ....   Date...

Exercise	Sets	Reps	Weight	PR

Cardio	Time	Distance	Intensity	PR

Supplements...
....

Comments ....
....
....

things to improve .... things to try out...
....

WORKOUT ....   Date...................................

Exercise	Sets	Reps	Weight	PR

Cardio	Time	Distance	Intensity	PR

Supplements...
....

Comments ....
....
....

things to improve .... things to try out.......................................
....

WORKOUT .... Date ....

Exercise	Sets	Reps	Weight	PR

Cardio	Time	Distance	Intensity	PR

Supplements ....
....

Comments ....
....
....

things to improve ....   things to try out ....
....

WORKOUT ....   Date.................................

Exercise	Sets	Reps	Weight	PR

Cardio	Time	Distance	Intensity	PR

Supplements...
....

Comments ....
....
....

things to improve ....   things to try out.......................................
....

WORKOUT .... Date.................................

Exercise	Sets	Reps	Weight	PR

Cardio	Time	Distance	Intensity	PR

Supplements...
....

Comments ....
....
....

things to improve ....   things to try out...
....

WORKOUT ....   Date..................................

Exercise	Sets	Reps	Weight	PR

Cardio	Time	Distance	Intensity	PR

Supplements..
....

Comments ....
....
....

things to improve ....   things to try out..
....

WORKOUT ....   Date...

Exercise	Sets	Reps	Weight	PR

Cardio	Time	Distance	Intensity	PR

Supplements...
....

Comments ....
....
....

things to improve ....   things to try out...
....

WORKOUT ....   Date...............................

Exercise	Sets	Reps	Weight	PR

Cardio	Time	Distance	Intensity	PR

Supplements...
....

Comments ....
....
....

things to improve ....   things to try out...
....

WORKOUT .... Date...................................

Exercise	Sets	Reps	Weight	PR

Cardio	Time	Distance	Intensity	PR

Supplements..

....

Comments ....

....

....

things to improve .... things to try out..............................

....

WORKOUT ....   Date.....................................

Exercise	Sets	Reps	Weight	PR

Cardio	Time	Distance	Intensity	PR

Supplements..
....

Comments ....
....
....

things to improve ....   things to try out..........................
....

WORKOUT ....   Date................................

Exercise	Sets	Reps	Weight	PR

Cardio	Time	Distance	Intensity	PR

Supplements...
....

Comments ....
....
....

things to improve ....   things to try out.................................
....

WORKOUT ....   Date....................................

Exercise	Sets	Reps	Weight	PR

Cardio	Time	Distance	Intensity	PR

Supplements...
....

Comments ....
....
....

things to improve ....   things to try out...
....

WORKOUT .... Date ....

Exercise	Sets	Reps	Weight	PR

Cardio	Time	Distance	Intensity	PR

Supplements ....
....

Comments ....
....
....

things to improve .... things to try out ....
....

WORKOUT ....   Date.................................

Exercise	Sets	Reps	Weight	PR

Cardio	Time	Distance	Intensity	PR

Supplements...
....

Comments ....
....
....

things to improve ....   things to try out......................................
....

WORKOUT ....   Date................................

Exercise	Sets	Reps	Weight	PR

Cardio	Time	Distance	Intensity	PR

Supplements...
....

Comments ....
....
....

things to improve ....   things to try out.......................................
....

WORKOUT ....   Date...

Exercise	Sets	Reps	Weight	PR

Cardio	Time	Distance	Intensity	PR

Supplements...
....

Comments ....
....
....

things to improve ....   things to try out....................................
....

WORKOUT ....   Date..

Exercise	Sets	Reps	Weight	PR

Cardio	Time	Distance	Intensity	PR

Supplements...
....

Comments ....
....
....

things to improve ....   things to try out...
....

WORKOUT ....   Date.................................

Exercise	Sets	Reps	Weight	PR

Cardio	Time	Distance	Intensity	PR

Supplements...
....

Comments ....
....
....

things to improve ....   things to try out...............................
....

WORKOUT ....   Date...

Exercise	Sets	Reps	Weight	PR

Cardio	Time	Distance	Intensity	PR

Supplements..

....

Comments ....

....

....

things to improve ....   things to try out...

....

WORKOUT .... Date................................

Exercise	Sets	Reps	Weight	PR

Cardio	Time	Distance	Intensity	PR

Supplements...
....

Comments ....
....
....

things to improve .... things to try out..................................
....

WORKOUT ....   Date..

Exercise	Sets	Reps	Weight	PR

Cardio	Time	Distance	Intensity	PR

Supplements...

....

Comments ....

....

....

things to improve .... things to try out...

....

WORKOUT ....   Date.................................

Exercise	Sets	Reps	Weight	PR

Cardio	Time	Distance	Intensity	PR

Supplements..
....

Comments ....
....
....

things to improve ....   things to try out......................................
....

WORKOUT ....   Date..

Exercise	Sets	Reps	Weight	PR

Cardio	Time	Distance	Intensity	PR

Supplements..
....

Comments ....
....
....

things to improve ....   things to try out..
....

WORKOUT .... Date...................................

Exercise	Sets	Reps	Weight	PR

Cardio	Time	Distance	Intensity	PR

Supplements...
....

Comments ....
....
....

things to improve .... things to try out...................................
....

WORKOUT .... Date................................

Exercise	Sets	Reps	Weight	PR

Cardio	Time	Distance	Intensity	PR

Supplements...

....

Comments ....

....

....

things to improve ....   things to try out...

....

WORKOUT .... Date.....................................

Exercise	Sets	Reps	Weight	PR

Cardio	Time	Distance	Intensity	PR

Supplements...
....

Comments ....
....
....

things to improve .... things to try out..............................
....

WORKOUT .... Date.................................

Exercise	Sets	Reps	Weight	PR

Cardio	Time	Distance	Intensity	PR

Supplements..
....

Comments ....
....
....

things to improve .... things to try out.................................
....

WORKOUT ....   Date..................................

Exercise	Sets	Reps	Weight	PR

Cardio	Time	Distance	Intensity	PR

Supplements..

....

Comments ....

....

....

things to improve ....   things to try out..

....

WORKOUT ....   Date................................

Exercise	Sets	Reps	Weight	PR

Cardio	Time	Distance	Intensity	PR

Supplements..

....

Comments ....

....

....

things to improve ....   things to try out................................

....

Workout ....   Date................................

Exercise	Sets	Reps	Weight	PR

Cardio	Time	Distance	Intensity	PR

Supplements..
....

Comments ....
....
....

things to improve ....   things to try out..............................
....

WORKOUT .... Date...

Exercise	Sets	Reps	Weight	PR

Cardio	Time	Distance	Intensity	PR

Supplements...
....

Comments ....
....
....

things to improve .... things to try out..........................
....

WORKOUT ....   Date...................................

Exercise	Sets	Reps	Weight	PR

Cardio	Time	Distance	Intensity	PR

Supplements..
....

Comments ....
....
....

things to improve ....   things to try out...
....

WORKOUT .... Date ....

Exercise	Sets	Reps	Weight	PR

Cardio	Time	Distance	Intensity	PR

Supplements ....
....

Comments ....
....
....

things to improve .... things to try out ....
....

WORKOUT ....   Date.................................

Exercise	Sets	Reps	Weight	PR

Cardio	Time	Distance	Intensity	PR

Supplements..
....

Comments ....
....
....

things to improve .... things to try out...........................
....

WORKOUT .... Date...

Exercise	Sets	Reps	Weight	PR

Cardio	Time	Distance	Intensity	PR

Supplements...
....

Comments ....
....
....

things to improve .... things to try out...
....

WORKOUT ....   Date.................................

Exercise	Sets	Reps	Weight	PR

Cardio	Time	Distance	Intensity	PR

Supplements..

....

Comments ....

....

....

things to improve ....   things to try out...

....

WORKOUT .... Date................................

Exercise	Sets	Reps	Weight	PR

Cardio	Time	Distance	Intensity	PR

Supplements..

....

Comments ....

....

....

things to improve ....   things to try out..

....

WORKOUT .... Date..................................

Exercise	Sets	Reps	Weight	PR

Cardio	Time	Distance	Intensity	PR

Supplements...
....

Comments ....
....
....

things to improve .... things to try out.................................
....

WORKOUT .... Date...

Exercise	Sets	Reps	Weight	PR

Cardio	Time	Distance	Intensity	PR

Supplements...

....

Comments ....

....

....

things to improve .... things to try out..

....

WORKOUT ....   Date.....................................

Exercise	Sets	Reps	Weight	PR

Cardio	Time	Distance	Intensity	PR

Supplements...
....

Comments ....
....
....

things to improve ....   things to try out...
....

WORKOUT .... Date...

Exercise	Sets	Reps	Weight	PR

Cardio	Time	Distance	Intensity	PR

Supplements...
....

Comments ....
....
....

things to improve .... things to try out.......................................
....

WORKOUT

Workout ....   Date...................................

Exercise	Sets	Reps	Weight	PR

Cardio	Time	Distance	Intensity	PR

Supplements...
....

Comments ....
....
....

things to improve ....   things to try out...................................
....

WORKOUT .... Date ....

Exercise	Sets	Reps	Weight	PR

Cardio	Time	Distance	Intensity	PR

Supplements ....
....

Comments ....
....
....

things to improve .... things to try out ....
....

WORKOUT ....   Date ....

Exercise	Sets	Reps	Weight	PR

Cardio	Time	Distance	Intensity	PR

Supplements...
....

Comments ....
....
....

things to improve ....   things to try out ....
....

WORKOUT ....   Date..................................

Exercise	Sets	Reps	Weight	PR

Cardio	Time	Distance	Intensity	PR

Supplements..
....

Comments ....
....
....

things to improve ....   things to try out..............................
....

WORKOUT .... Date ....

Exercise	Sets	Reps	Weight	PR

Cardio	Time	Distance	Intensity	PR

Supplements ....
....

Comments ....
....
....

things to improve .... things to try out...............................
....

WORKOUT ....   Date...................................

Exercise	Sets	Reps	Weight	PR

Cardio	Time	Distance	Intensity	PR

Supplements...

....

Comments ....

....

....

things to improve ....   things to try out...........................

....

WORKOUT ....   Date...................................

Exercise	Sets	Reps	Weight	PR

Cardio	Time	Distance	Intensity	PR

Supplements..
....

Comments ....
....
....

things to improve ....   things to try out...
....

WORKOUT ....   Date..

Exercise	Sets	Reps	Weight	PR

Cardio	Time	Distance	Intensity	PR

Supplements..
....

Comments ....
....
....

things to improve ....   things to try out.....................................
....

WORKOUT ....   Date.................................

Exercise	Sets	Reps	Weight	PR

Cardio	Time	Distance	Intensity	PR

Supplements...
....

Comments ....
....
....

things to improve ....   things to try out.................................
....

WORKOUT .... Date..

Exercise	Sets	Reps	Weight	PR

Cardio	Time	Distance	Intensity	PR

Supplements...
....

Comments ....
....
....

things to improve .... things to try out..
....

WORKOUT .... Date...............................

Exercise	Sets	Reps	Weight	PR

Cardio	Time	Distance	Intensity	PR

Supplements...
....

Comments ....
....
....

things to improve .... things to try out..
....

WORKOUT ....   Date...................................

Exercise	Sets	Reps	Weight	PR

Cardio	Time	Distance	Intensity	PR

Supplements...
....

Comments ....
....
....

things to improve ....   things to try out..
....

WORKOUT .... Date...................................

Exercise	Sets	Reps	Weight	PR

Cardio	Time	Distance	Intensity	PR

Supplements..
....

Comments ....
....
....

things to improve .... things to try out...............................
....

WORKOUT ....   Date..

Exercise	Sets	Reps	Weight	PR

Cardio	Time	Distance	Intensity	PR

Supplements..
....

Comments ....
....
....

things to improve ....   things to try out...
....

Workout ....   Date..................................

Exercise	Sets	Reps	Weight	PR

Cardio	Time	Distance	Intensity	PR

Supplements..
....

Comments ....
....
....

things to improve .... things to try out...................................
....

WORKOUT .... Date ....

Exercise	Sets	Reps	Weight	PR

Cardio	Time	Distance	Intensity	PR

supplements ....
....

Comments ....
....
....

things to improve .... things to try out ....
....

WORKOUT ....   Date.......................................

Exercise	Sets	Reps	Weight	PR

Cardio	Time	Distance	Intensity	PR

Supplements...
....

Comments ....
....
....

things to improve ....   things to try out...
....

WORKOUT ....   Date..

Exercise	Sets	Reps	Weight	PR

Cardio	Time	Distance	Intensity	PR

Supplements...
....

Comments ....
....
....

things to improve ....   things to try out...
....

WORKOUT ....   Date...................................

Exercise	Sets	Reps	Weight	PR

Cardio	Time	Distance	Intensity	PR

Supplements..
....

Comments ....
....
....

things to improve ....   things to try out ....
....

WORKOUT .... Date..

Exercise	Sets	Reps	Weight	PR

Cardio	Time	Distance	Intensity	PR

Supplements..
....

Comments ....
....
....

things to improve .... things to try out..
....

WORKOUT ....   Date.......................................

Exercise	Sets	Reps	Weight	PR

Cardio	Time	Distance	Intensity	PR

Supplements..
....

Comments ....
....
....

things to improve ....   things to try out..
....

WORKOUT ....   Date...................................

Exercise	Sets	Reps	Weight	PR

Cardio	Time	Distance	Intensity	PR

Supplements...
....

Comments ....
....
....

things to improve ....   things to try out...........................
....

WORKOUT

Workout ....   Date ....

Exercise	Sets	Reps	Weight	PR

Cardio	Time	Distance	Intensity	PR

Supplements ....
....

Comments ....
....
....

things to improve ....   things to try out ....
....

WORKOUT ....   Date...

Exercise	Sets	Reps	Weight	PR

Cardio	Time	Distance	Intensity	PR

Supplements..
....

Comments ....
....
....

things to improve ....   things to try out...
....

WORKOUT ....   Date.......................................

Exercise	Sets	Reps	Weight	PR

Cardio	Time	Distance	Intensity	PR

Supplements...
....

Comments ....
....
....

things to improve .... things to try out...
....

WORKOUT ....   Date...

Exercise	Sets	Reps	Weight	PR

Cardio	Time	Distance	Intensity	PR

Supplements...
....

Comments ....
....
....

things to improve ....   things to try out...
....

WORKOUT ....   Date................................

Exercise	Sets	Reps	Weight	PR

Cardio	Time	Distance	Intensity	PR

Supplements..
....

Comments ....
....
....

things to improve ....   things to try out...............................
....

Workout ....   Date...

Exercise	Sets	Reps	Weight	PR

Cardio	Time	Distance	Intensity	PR

Supplements...
....

Comments ....
....
....

things to improve ....   things to try out...
....

WORKOUT .... Date...............................

Exercise	Sets	Reps	Weight	PR

Cardio	Time	Distance	Intensity	PR

Supplements...
....

Comments ....
....
....

things to improve .... things to try out...............................
....

WORKOUT .... Date................................

Exercise	Sets	Reps	Weight	PR

Cardio	Time	Distance	Intensity	PR

Supplements..
....

Comments ....
....
....

things to improve .... things to try out........................
....

WORKOUT .... Date................................

Exercise	Sets	Reps	Weight	PR

Cardio	Time	Distance	Intensity	PR

Supplements...
....

Comments ....
....
....

things to improve .... things to try out................................
....

WORKOUT .... Date....................................

Exercise	Sets	Reps	Weight	PR

Cardio	Time	Distance	Intensity	PR

Supplements...

....

Comments ....

....

....

things to improve .... things to try out..

....

WORKOUT ....   Date.................................

Exercise	Sets	Reps	Weight	PR

Cardio	Time	Distance	Intensity	PR

Supplements...
....

Comments ....
....
....

things to improve ....   things to try out...............................
....

WORKOUT ....   Date..

Exercise	Sets	Reps	Weight	PR

Cardio	Time	Distance	Intensity	PR

Supplements..
....

Comments ....
....
....

things to improve ....   things to try out..
....

WORKOUT .... Date..................................

Exercise	Sets	Reps	Weight	PR

Cardio	Time	Distance	Intensity	PR

Supplements...
....

Comments ....
....
....

things to improve .... things to try out..
....

WORKOUT .... Date..

Exercise	Sets	Reps	Weight	PR

Cardio	Time	Distance	Intensity	PR

Supplements..
....

Comments ....
....
....

things to improve .... things to try out..
....

WORKOUT ....   Date.....................................

Exercise	Sets	Reps	Weight	PR

Cardio	Time	Distance	Intensity	PR

Supplements...
....

Comments ....
....
....

things to improve .... things to try out...
....

WORKOUT .... Date..

Exercise	Sets	Reps	Weight	PR

Cardio	Time	Distance	Intensity	PR

Supplements...
....

Comments ....
....
....

things to improve .... things to try out...
....

WORKOUT ....   Date.................................

Exercise	Sets	Reps	Weight	PR

Cardio	Time	Distance	Intensity	PR

Supplements..
....

Comments ....
....
....

things to improve .... things to try out.............................
....

WORKOUT ....   Date ....

Exercise	Sets	Reps	Weight	PR

Cardio	Time	Distance	Intensity	PR

Supplements ....

....

Comments ....

....

....

things to improve ....   things to try out ....

....

Workout ....   Date...

Exercise	Sets	Reps	Weight	PR

Cardio	Time	Distance	Intensity	PR

Supplements...
....

Comments ....
....
....

things to improve ....   things to try out...
....

WORKOUT ....   Date...................................

Exercise	Sets	Reps	Weight	PR

Cardio	Time	Distance	Intensity	PR

Supplements...
....

Comments ....
....
....

things to improve ....   things to try out..................................
....

WORKOUT .... Date................................

Exercise	Sets	Reps	Weight	PR

Cardio	Time	Distance	Intensity	PR

Supplements...
....

Comments ....
....
....

things to improve .... things to try out...
....

WORKOUT .... Date.................................

Exercise	Sets	Reps	Weight	PR

Cardio	Time	Distance	Intensity	PR

Supplements...
....

Comments ....
....
....

things to improve .... things to try out.................................
....

WORKOUT ....   Date......................................

Exercise	Sets	Reps	Weight	PR

Cardio	Time	Distance	Intensity	PR

Supplements...
....

Comments ....
....
....

things to improve ....   things to try out..................................
....

WORKOUT .... Date...................................

Exercise	Sets	Reps	Weight	PR

Cardio	Time	Distance	Intensity	PR

Supplements...
....

Comments ....
....
....

things to improve .... things to try out...
....

WORKOUT ....   Date...................................

Exercise	Sets	Reps	Weight	PR

Cardio	Time	Distance	Intensity	PR

Supplements...
....

Comments ....
....
....

things to improve ....   things to try out...
....

Workout .... Date..................................

Exercise	Sets	Reps	Weight	PR

Cardio	Time	Distance	Intensity	PR

Supplements..

....

Comments ....

....

....

things to improve ....   things to try out.......................................

....

WORKOUT .... Date.................................

Exercise	Sets	Reps	Weight	PR

Cardio	Time	Distance	Intensity	PR

Supplements...

....

Comments ....

....

....

things to improve .... things to try out............................

....

WORKOUT ....   Date...................................

Exercise	Sets	Reps	Weight	PR

Cardio	Time	Distance	Intensity	PR

Supplements...
....

Comments ....
....
....

things to improve ....   things to try out.................................
....

WORKOUT ....   Date...............................

Exercise	Sets	Reps	Weight	PR

Cardio	Time	Distance	Intensity	PR

Supplements..

....

Comments ....

....

....

things to improve ....   things to try out...............................

....

WORKOUT ....   Date......................................

Exercise	Sets	Reps	Weight	PR

Cardio	Time	Distance	Intensity	PR

Supplements..
....

Comments ....
....
....

things to improve ....   things to try out...
....

Workout .... Date.................................

Exercise	Sets	Reps	Weight	PR

Cardio	Time	Distance	Intensity	PR

Supplements...
....

Comments ....
....
....

things to improve .... things to try out......................................
....

WORKOUT .... Date...........................

Exercise	Sets	Reps	Weight	PR

Cardio	Time	Distance	Intensity	PR

Supplements...
....

Comments ....
....
....

things to improve .... things to try out............................
....

WORKOUT ....　　　　Date...................................

Exercise	Sets	Reps	Weight	PR

Cardio	Time	Distance	Intensity	PR

Supplements..
....

Comments ....
....
....

things to improve .... things to try out...............................
....

WORKOUT .... Date ....

Exercise	Sets	Reps	Weight	PR

Cardio	Time	Distance	Intensity	PR

Supplements ....
....

Comments ....
....
....

things to improve .... things to try out ....
....

Workout ....   Date ....

Exercise	Sets	Reps	Weight	PR

Cardio	Time	Distance	Intensity	PR

Supplements...
....

Comments ....
....
....

things to improve ....   things to try out.............................
....

WORKOUT ....   Date...

Exercise	Sets	Reps	Weight	PR

Cardio	Time	Distance	Intensity	PR

Supplements...
....

Comments ....
....
....

things to improve ....   things to try out..
....

WORKOUT .... Date............................

Exercise	Sets	Reps	Weight	PR

Cardio	Time	Distance	Intensity	PR

Supplements..
....

Comments ....
....
....

things to improve .... things to try out.............................
....

WORKOUT .... Date....................................

Exercise	Sets	Reps	Weight	PR

Cardio	Time	Distance	Intensity	PR

Supplements...

....

Comments ....

....

....

things to improve .... things to try out...............................

....

Workout .... Date...............................

Exercise	Sets	Reps	Weight	PR

Cardio	Time	Distance	Intensity	PR

Supplements...
....

Comments ....
....
....

things to improve ....   things to try out.....................................
....

WORKOUT .... Date....................................

Exercise	Sets	Reps	Weight	PR

Cardio	Time	Distance	Intensity	PR

Supplements...

....

Comments ....

....

....

things to improve .... things to try out...............................

....

Workout .... Date................................

Exercise	Sets	Reps	Weight	PR

Cardio	Time	Distance	Intensity	PR

Supplements..
....

Comments ....
....
....

things to improve .... things to try out...
....

WORKOUT .... Date ....

Exercise	Sets	Reps	Weight	PR

Cardio	Time	Distance	Intensity	PR

Supplements ....
....

Comments ....
....
....

things to improve .... things to try out ....
....

Workout ....   Date ....

Exercise	Sets	Reps	Weight	PR

Cardio	Time	Distance	Intensity	PR

Supplements ....
....

Comments ....
....
....

things to improve ....   things to try out ....
....

WORKOUT .... Date..

Exercise	Sets	Reps	Weight	PR

Cardio	Time	Distance	Intensity	PR

Supplements...

....

Comments ....

....

....

things to improve .... things to try out.................................

....

Workout ....   Date....................................

Exercise	Sets	Reps	Weight	PR

Cardio	Time	Distance	Intensity	PR

Supplements..
....

Comments ....
....
....

things to improve .... things to try out...
....

WORKOUT ....   Date...

Exercise	Sets	Reps	Weight	PR

Cardio	Time	Distance	Intensity	PR

Supplements...
....

Comments ....
....
....

things to improve ....   things to try out...
....

WORKOUT ....　　　Date...

Exercise	Sets	Reps	Weight	PR

Cardio	Time	Distance	Intensity	PR

Supplements...
....

Comments ....
....
....

things to improve ....　things to try out...
....　...

WORKOUT .... Date ....

Exercise	Sets	Reps	Weight	PR

Cardio	Time	Distance	Intensity	PR

Supplements ....
....

Comments ....
....
....

things to improve .... things to try out ....
....

WORKOUT ....   Date...................................

Exercise	Sets	Reps	Weight	PR

Cardio	Time	Distance	Intensity	PR

Supplements..
....

Comments ....
....
....

things to improve ....   things to try out......................................
....

WORKOUT .... Date.......................................

Exercise	Sets	Reps	Weight	PR

Cardio	Time	Distance	Intensity	PR

Supplements..
....

Comments ....
....
....

things to improve ....   things to try out...
....

WORKOUT .... Date.................................

Exercise	Sets	Reps	Weight	PR

Cardio	Time	Distance	Intensity	PR

Supplements..
....

Comments ....
....
....

things to improve ....   things to try out...
....

WORKOUT .... Date...........................

Exercise	Sets	Reps	Weight	PR

Cardio	Time	Distance	Intensity	PR

Supplements...

....

Comments ....

....

....

things to improve .... things to try out............................

....

WORKOUT .... Date..................................

Exercise	Sets	Reps	Weight	PR

Cardio	Time	Distance	Intensity	PR

Supplements...
....

Comments ....
....
....

things to improve .... things to try out..
....

WORKOUT ....   Date..

Exercise	Sets	Reps	Weight	PR

Cardio	Time	Distance	Intensity	PR

Supplements..
....

Comments ....
....
....

things to improve ....   things to try out...
....

Workout ....   Date..................................

Exercise	Sets	Reps	Weight	PR

Cardio	Time	Distance	Intensity	PR

Supplements..
....

Comments ....
....
....

things to improve ....   things to try out...........................
....

WORKOUT ....   Date...................................

Exercise	Sets	Reps	Weight	PR

Cardio	Time	Distance	Intensity	PR

Supplements..
....

Comments ....
....
....

things to improve .... things to try out.................................
....

WORKOUT .... Date................................

Exercise	Sets	Reps	Weight	PR

Cardio	Time	Distance	Intensity	PR

Supplements..
....

Comments ....
....
....

things to improve .... things to try out..............................
....

WORKOUT ....   Date..

Exercise	Sets	Reps	Weight	PR

Cardio	Time	Distance	Intensity	PR

Supplements..
....

Comments ....
....
....

things to improve ....   things to try out...
....

WORKOUT ....   Date...................................

Exercise	Sets	Reps	Weight	PR

Cardio	Time	Distance	Intensity	PR

Supplements..
....

Comments ....
....
....

things to improve ....   things to try out...............................
....

WORKOUT .... Date...

Exercise	Sets	Reps	Weight	PR

Cardio	Time	Distance	Intensity	PR

Supplements...
....

Comments ....
....
....

things to improve .... things to try out..
....

WORKOUT ....   Date...................................

Exercise	Sets	Reps	Weight	PR

Cardio	Time	Distance	Intensity	PR

Supplements...
....

Comments ....
....
....

things to improve ....   things to try out.....................................
....

WORKOUT ....   Date..

Exercise	Sets	Reps	Weight	PR

Cardio	Time	Distance	Intensity	PR

Supplements..

....

Comments ....

....

....

things to improve ....   things to try out...

....

WORKOUT ....   Date..

Exercise	Sets	Reps	Weight	PR

Cardio	Time	Distance	Intensity	PR

Supplements..

....

Comments ....

....

....

things to improve ....   things to try out..

....

WORKOUT .... Date...

Exercise	Sets	Reps	Weight	PR

Cardio	Time	Distance	Intensity	PR

Supplements...
....

Comments ....
....
....

things to improve .... things to try out...
....

WORKOUT ....   Date..................................

Exercise	Sets	Reps	Weight	PR

Cardio	Time	Distance	Intensity	PR

Supplements..
....

Comments ....
....
....

things to improve ....   things to try out...............................
....

WORKOUT ....   Date................................

Exercise	Sets	Reps	Weight	PR

Cardio	Time	Distance	Intensity	PR

Supplements..

....

Comments ....

....

....

things to improve ....   things to try out..

....

Workout ....   Date.....................................

Exercise	Sets	Reps	Weight	PR

Cardio	Time	Distance	Intensity	PR

Supplements..
....

Comments ....
....
....

things to improve ....   things to try out..
....

WORKOUT ....   Date..

Exercise	Sets	Reps	Weight	PR

Cardio	Time	Distance	Intensity	PR

Supplements..

....

Comments ....

....

....

things to improve ....   things to try out..

....

Workout

Workout ....   Date ....

Exercise	Sets	Reps	Weight	PR

Cardio	Time	Distance	Intensity	PR

Supplements ....
....

Comments ....
....
....

things to improve ....   things to try out ....
....

WORKOUT .... Date.................................

Exercise	Sets	Reps	Weight	PR

Cardio	Time	Distance	Intensity	PR

Supplements...
....

Comments ....
....
....

things to improve .... things to try out..............................
....

WORKOUT .... Date..

Exercise	Sets	Reps	Weight	PR

Cardio	Time	Distance	Intensity	PR

Supplements...
....

Comments ....
....
....

things to improve ....   things to try out...
....

WORKOUT ....   Date..

Exercise	Sets	Reps	Weight	PR

Cardio	Time	Distance	Intensity	PR

Supplements...

....

Comments ....

....

....

things to improve ....   things to try out.................................

....

Workout ....   Date................................

Exercise	Sets	Reps	Weight	PR

Cardio	Time	Distance	Intensity	PR

Supplements...
....

Comments ....
....
....

things to improve ....   things to try out.................................
....

WORKOUT .... Date.................................

Exercise	Sets	Reps	Weight	PR

Cardio	Time	Distance	Intensity	PR

Supplements...
....

Comments ....
....
....

things to improve .... things to try out...........................
....

WORKOUT ....   Date...................................

Exercise	Sets	Reps	Weight	PR

Cardio	Time	Distance	Intensity	PR

Supplements...
....

Comments ....
....
....

things to improve ....   things to try out...
....

WORKOUT .... Date.................................

Exercise	Sets	Reps	Weight	PR

Cardio	Time	Distance	Intensity	PR

Supplements..
....

Comments ....
....
....

things to improve .... things to try out.................................
....

WORKOUT .... Date....................................

Exercise	Sets	Reps	Weight	PR

Cardio	Time	Distance	Intensity	PR

Supplements..
....

Comments ....
....
....

things to improve .... things to try out...
....

WORKOUT ....   Date...................................

Exercise	Sets	Reps	Weight	PR

Cardio	Time	Distance	Intensity	PR

Supplements...
....

Comments ....
....
....

things to improve ....   things to try out...
....

WORKOUT ....   Date.....................................

Exercise	Sets	Reps	Weight	PR

Cardio	Time	Distance	Intensity	PR

Supplements...
....

Comments ....
....
....

things to improve ....   things to try out..
....

WORKOUT .... Date...

Exercise	Sets	Reps	Weight	PR

Cardio	Time	Distance	Intensity	PR

Supplements...
....

Comments ....
....
....

things to improve .... things to try out...
....

Workout ....   Date...................................

Exercise	Sets	Reps	Weight	PR

Cardio	Time	Distance	Intensity	PR

Supplements...
....

Comments ....
....
....

things to improve ....   things to try out ....
....

WORKOUT .... Date...

Exercise	Sets	Reps	Weight	PR

Cardio	Time	Distance	Intensity	PR

Supplements...

....

Comments ....

....

....

things to improve ....   things to try out...

....

Workout ....   Date................................

Exercise	Sets	Reps	Weight	PR

Cardio	Time	Distance	Intensity	PR

Supplements...
....

Comments ....
....
....

things to improve ....   things to try out.........................
....

WORKOUT .... Date.................................

Exercise	Sets	Reps	Weight	PR

Cardio	Time	Distance	Intensity	PR

Supplements...
....

Comments ....
....
....

things to improve .... things to try out....................................
....

WORKOUT ....   Date...................................

Exercise	Sets	Reps	Weight	PR

Cardio	Time	Distance	Intensity	PR

Supplements...
....

Comments ....
....
....

things to improve ....   things to try out.....................................
....

WORKOUT .... Date..

Exercise	Sets	Reps	Weight	PR

Cardio	Time	Distance	Intensity	PR

Supplements..
....

Comments ....
....
....

things to improve .... things to try out..
....

WORKOUT .... Date.......................................

Exercise	Sets	Reps	Weight	PR

Cardio	Time	Distance	Intensity	PR

Supplements...
....

Comments ....
....
....

things to improve .... things to try out...................................
....

WORKOUT

Workout ....   Date.................................

Exercise	Sets	Reps	Weight	PR

Cardio	Time	Distance	Intensity	PR

Supplements..
....

Comments ....
....
....

things to improve ....   things to try out.......................
....

WORKOUT ....   Date...................................

Exercise	Sets	Reps	Weight	PR

Cardio	Time	Distance	Intensity	PR

Supplements..
....

Comments ....
....
....

things to improve......................................   things to try out...
....

WORKOUT .... Date................................

Exercise	Sets	Reps	Weight	PR

Cardio	Time	Distance	Intensity	PR

Supplements..
....

Comments ....
....
....

things to improve .... things to try out...............................
....

WORKOUT ....　　Date.................................

Exercise	Sets	Reps	Weight	PR

Cardio	Time	Distance	Intensity	PR

Supplements...
....

Comments ....
....
....

things to improve..　things to try out.................................
....　...

WORKOUT ....   Date..

Exercise		Sets	Reps	Weight	PR

Cardio		Time	Distance	Intensity	PR

Supplements...
....

Comments ....
....
....

things to improve ....   things to try out...
....

WORKOUT ....   Date.....................................

Exercise	Sets	Reps	Weight	PR

Cardio	Time	Distance	Intensity	PR

Supplements..
....

Comments ....
....
....

things to improve ....   things to try out..
....

WORKOUT .... Date...

Exercise	Sets	Reps	Weight	PR

Cardio	Time	Distance	Intensity	PR

Supplements...
....

Comments ....
....
....

things to improve .... things to try out...............................
....

WORKOUT

Workout ....   Date.....................................

Exercise	Sets	Reps	Weight	PR

Cardio	Time	Distance	Intensity	PR

Supplements...
....

Comments ....
....
....

things to improve ....   things to try out................................
....

WORKOUT ....   Date...

Exercise	Sets	Reps	Weight	PR

Cardio	Time	Distance	Intensity	PR

Supplements...
....

Comments ....
....
....

things to improve ....   things to try out..
....

WORKOUT ....   Date.......................................

Exercise	Sets	Reps	Weight	PR

Cardio	Time	Distance	Intensity	PR

Supplements...
....

Comments ....
....
....

things to improve ....   things to try out.......................................
....

WORKOUT .... Date...

Exercise	Sets	Reps	Weight	PR

Cardio	Time	Distance	Intensity	PR

Supplements...
....

Comments ....
....
....

things to improve .... things to try out...
....

WORKOUT ....   Date...............................

Exercise	Sets	Reps	Weight	PR

Cardio	Time	Distance	Intensity	PR

Supplements..
....

Comments ....
....
....

things to improve ....   things to try out..
....

WORKOUT .... Date...

Exercise	Sets	Reps	Weight	PR

Cardio	Time	Distance	Intensity	PR

Supplements...
....

Comments ....
....
....

things to improve .... things to try out...................................
....

WORKOUT

Workout .... Date.....................................

Exercise	Sets	Reps	Weight	PR

Cardio	Time	Distance	Intensity	PR

Supplements...
....

Comments ....
....
....

things to improve ....   things to try out..........................
....

WORKOUT ....   Date...................................

Exercise	Sets	Reps	Weight	PR

Cardio	Time	Distance	Intensity	PR

Supplements...
....

Comments ....
....
....

things to improve ....   things to try out...
....

WORKOUT .... Date...................................

Exercise	Sets	Reps	Weight	PR

Cardio	Time	Distance	Intensity	PR

Supplements...
....

Comments ....
....
....

things to improve .... things to try out.................................
....

WORKOUT .... Date..

Exercise	Sets	Reps	Weight	PR

Cardio	Time	Distance	Intensity	PR

Supplements...
....

Comments ....
....
....

things to improve .... things to try out..
....

Workout .... Date ....

Exercise	Sets	Reps	Weight	PR

Cardio	Time	Distance	Intensity	PR

Supplements ....
....

Comments ....
....
....

things to improve .... things to try out ....
....

WORKOUT .... Date................................

Exercise	Sets	Reps	Weight	PR

Cardio	Time	Distance	Intensity	PR

Supplements..
....

Comments ....
....
....

things to improve .... things to try out....................................
....

WORKOUT .... Date.....................................

Exercise	Sets	Reps	Weight	PR

Cardio	Time	Distance	Intensity	PR

Supplements..
....

Comments ....
....
....

things to improve .... things to try out...................................
....

WORKOUT .... Date..................................

Exercise	Sets	Reps	Weight	PR

Cardio	Time	Distance	Intensity	PR

Supplements..

....

Comments ....

....

....

things to improve .... things to try out..

....

WORKOUT ....   Date.................................

Exercise	Sets	Reps	Weight	PR

Cardio	Time	Distance	Intensity	PR

Supplements...
....

Comments ....
....
....

things to improve ....   things to try out.......................................
....

WORKOUT ....   Date.....................................

Exercise	Sets	Reps	Weight	PR

Cardio	Time	Distance	Intensity	PR

Supplements...
....

Comments ....
....
....

things to improve ....   things to try out...
....

WORKOUT .... Date...................................

Exercise	Sets	Reps	Weight	PR

Cardio	Time	Distance	Intensity	PR

Supplements..
....

Comments ....
....
....

things to improve .... things to try out...
....

WORKOUT ....   Date..

Exercise	Sets	Reps	Weight	PR

Cardio	Time	Distance	Intensity	PR

Supplements...
....

Comments ....
....
....

things to improve ....   things to try out...
....

WORKOUT .... Date ....

Exercise	Sets	Reps	Weight	PR

Cardio	Time	Distance	Intensity	PR

Supplements ....
....

Comments ....
....
....

things to improve .... things to try out ....
....

WORKOUT ....   Date..

Exercise	Sets	Reps	Weight	PR

Cardio	Time	Distance	Intensity	PR

Supplements...
....

Comments ....
....
....

things to improve ....   things to try out.......................................
....

WORKOUT .... Date..

Exercise	Sets	Reps	Weight	PR

Cardio	Time	Distance	Intensity	PR

Supplements..
....

Comments ....
....
....

things to improve .... things to try out...
....

| WORKOUT | .... | Date.. |

Exercise	Sets	Reps	Weight	PR

Cardio	Time	Distance	Intensity	PR

Supplements...

....

Comments ....

....

....

things to improve ....   things to try out...

....

WORKOUT .... Date................................

Exercise	Sets	Reps	Weight	PR

Cardio	Time	Distance	Intensity	PR

Supplements...
....

Comments ....
....
....

things to improve ....   things to try out...
....

WORKOUT ....   Date..

Exercise	Sets	Reps	Weight	PR

Cardio	Time	Distance	Intensity	PR

Supplements..
....

Comments ....
....
....

things to improve ....   things to try out..
....

Workout .... Date................................

Exercise	Sets	Reps	Weight	PR

Cardio	Time	Distance	Intensity	PR

Supplements..

....

Comments ....

....

....

things to improve .... things to try out...............................

....

WORKOUT .... Date.................................

Exercise	Sets	Reps	Weight	PR

Cardio	Time	Distance	Intensity	PR

Supplements...
....

Comments ....
....
....

things to improve ....   things to try out...
....

WORKOUT .... Date ....

Exercise	Sets	Reps	Weight	PR

Cardio	Time	Distance	Intensity	PR

Supplements ....
....

Comments ....
....
....

things to improve .... things to try out ....
....

WORKOUT .... Date.................................

Exercise		Sets	Reps	Weight	PR

Cardio		Time	Distance	Intensity	PR

Supplements...
....

Comments ....
....
....

things to improve .... things to try out...........................
....

WORKOUT .... Date..

Exercise	Sets	Reps	Weight	PR

Cardio	Time	Distance	Intensity	PR

Supplements...
....

Comments ....
....
....

things to improve .... things to try out.......................................
....

WORKOUT .... Date...................................

Exercise	Sets	Reps	Weight	PR

Cardio	Time	Distance	Intensity	PR

Supplements...
....

Comments ....
....
....

things to improve .... things to try out...
....

WORKOUT ....   Date.................................

Exercise	Sets	Reps	Weight	PR

Cardio	Time	Distance	Intensity	PR

Supplements..
....

Comments ....
....
....

things to improve ....   things to try out...............................
....

WORKOUT .... Date.................................

Exercise	Sets	Reps	Weight	PR

Cardio	Time	Distance	Intensity	PR

Supplements...
....

Comments ....
....
....

things to improve .... things to try out...............................
....

WORKOUT ....   Date...............................

Exercise	Sets	Reps	Weight	PR

Cardio	Time	Distance	Intensity	PR

Supplements..
....

Comments ....
....
....

things to improve ....   things to try out...
....

WORKOUT ....   Date..

Exercise	Sets	Reps	Weight	PR

Cardio	Time	Distance	Intensity	PR

Supplements...

....

Comments ....

....

....

things to improve .... things to try out...

....

Workout .... Date...

Exercise	Sets	Reps	Weight	PR

Cardio	Time	Distance	Intensity	PR

Supplements...
....

Comments ....
....
....

things to improve .... things to try out...............................
....

Workout .... Date...................................

Exercise	Sets	Reps	Weight	PR

Cardio	Time	Distance	Intensity	PR

Supplements...
....

Comments ....
....
....

things to improve .... things to try out...
....

WORKOUT

.... Date....................................

Exercise	Sets	Reps	Weight	PR

Cardio	Time	Distance	Intensity	PR

Supplements...
....

Comments ....
....
....

things to improve.................................... things to try out.............................
....

WORKOUT ....   Date.................................

Exercise	Sets	Reps	Weight	PR

Cardio	Time	Distance	Intensity	PR

Supplements...

....

Comments ....

....

....

things to improve ....   things to try out.................................

....

www.ingramcontent.com/pod-product-compliance
Lightning Source LLC
Chambersburg PA
CBHW080338290526

45790CB00010B/3745